TARA WAGNER

F*ck Cancer

This book was professionally typeset on Reedsy.
Find out more at reedsy.com

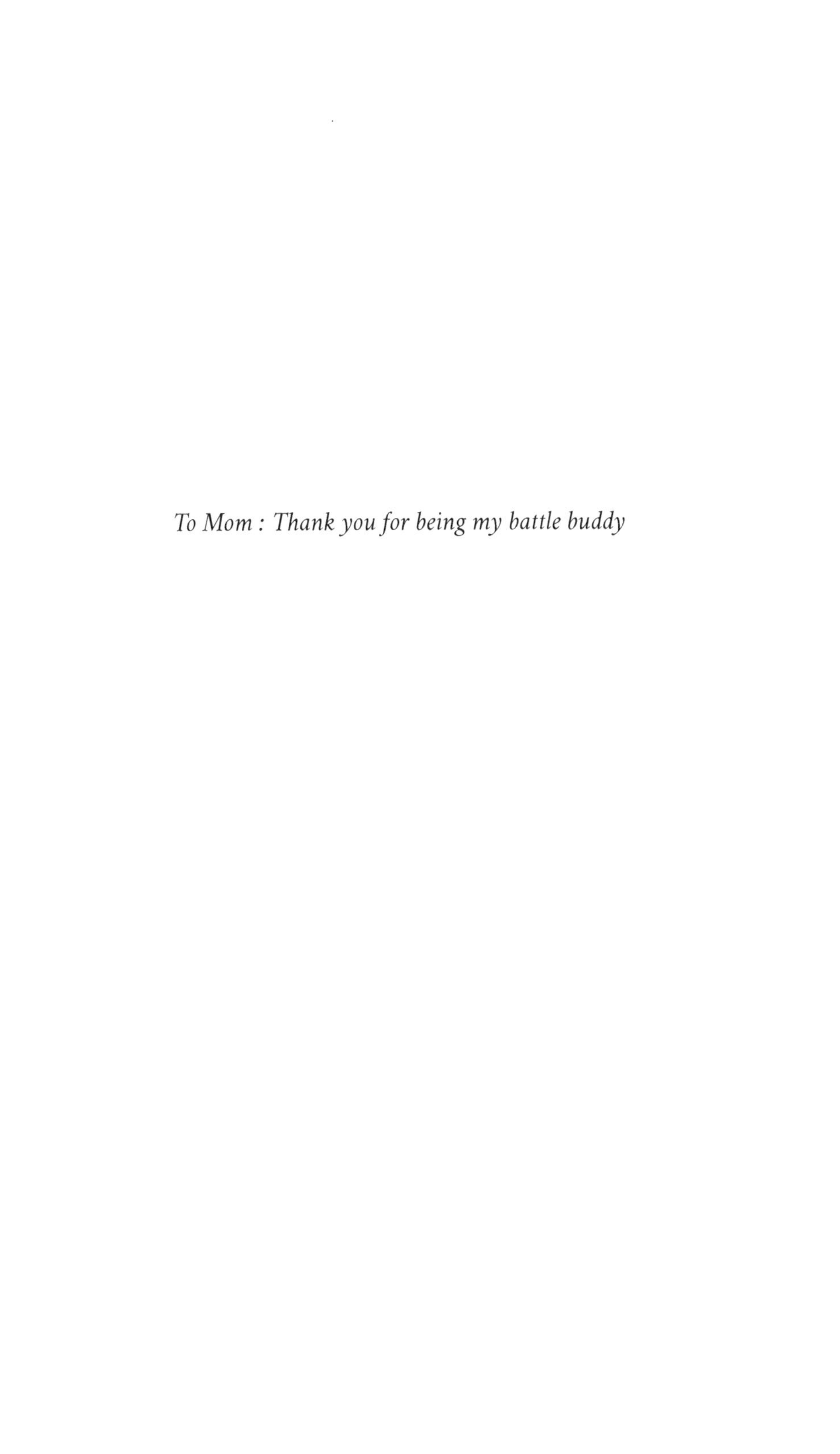

To Mom : Thank you for being my battle buddy

Contents

1

Introduction

I f you have anyone close to you that is fighting for their life, either family member or friend, cancer takes a toll on the quality of life. There will be many ups and downs along the way. Good days and bad days. Days that you will feel that you simply can not go on, and others that you can say with a resounding "I've Got This!"

This is my personal my personal journey discovering, being diagnosed, treating, and living with a grade 2 Astrocytoma [brain cancer]

I have been so blessed to have a strong support system surrounding me every step of the way.

A little backstory for me...I am a 42 year old divorced mother of two. I have a daughter-17 and a son-15. I am a full time,self-employed cosmetologist with a one chair salon in a small town in Nebraska. Long, busy days were the norm for me. I used to put in a lot of hours in the salon before I was diagnosed. The previous year, I had just gone through an extremely difficult divorce, But that's an entirely different story.

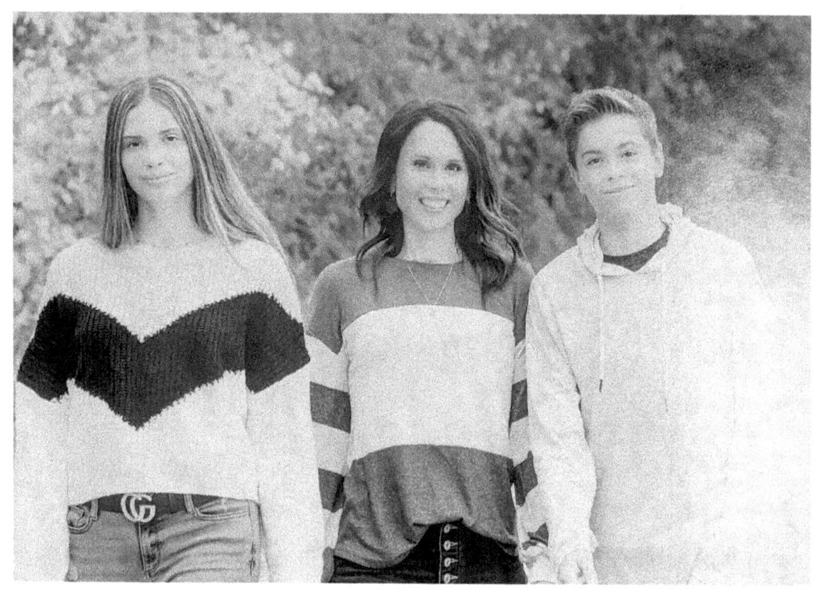

2

The Diagnosis

As previously mentioned, I had gone through a divorce. My ex carried the health insurance, so I had taken a part time job in the mornings at the UPS warehouse. It was going to take nine long months before I would qualify for health insurance, but I had my eye on the prize and I was determined to stick it out and make it work. It was the busy time of year at UPS and also at my salon. I was running myself ragged. My normally long days had now turned into 16 hour days six days a week. After a few months I started to not feel so great. I know what you're thinking, right? Duh, you can't keep that pace. That wasn't it though. I started to get dizzy, feeling nauseous, having constant headaches and pressure in my face, and the strangest nose bleeds. My daughter has had nose bleeds her entire life. These were not like that. I would have little blood clots come out when I blew my nose. I went to see my primary physician about it, and she explained to me that I could no longer put off the sinus surgery I was told I needed to have years before when I went to see an ear, nose and throat {ENT} doctor in Columbus. My doctor told me that if they did in-office cauterizing, she would do my entire nose. They didn't, so she had advised me not to even blow my nose or it would bleed.

I immediately got a hold of my mom and told her what was going on. She works at a hospital. She does credentialing and works closely with doctors, so she knows them on more of a personal level. I had resigned myself to needing to have sinus surgery, even though I was most definitely not looking forward to it. My mom recommended someone that she knew well and that she felt would do a good job. I made an appointment to drive the 2 hours one way to see him, since it would be closer to my parents. If I was going to have surgery I was going to need help and care.

My first appointment with the new ENT Dr. went ok, I thought. I told him everything that I had previously been told about needing sinus surgery, having a deviated septum and what not. He had asked if I could breathe through my nose, and I explained, kind of, through one side. I had always chalked it up to my deviated septum and allergies that I have. I also explained to him the pressure in my face, the bloody noses and the fact that I really couldn't smell anything anymore, unless it was very strong. He took an instrument that was long and skinny and looked up my nose. He then proceeded to tell me that he couldn't see any reason why I couldn't breathe. He said that there may be something that showed up on my CT inside my sinus cavity to explain what he couldn't see. He ordered a CT scan for me.

I made the trip back for the scan a couple of weeks later. I was at home when I got the call from the doctor that my scan was read by an Interventional Radiologist. He had seen a shadow and ordered an MRI, with and without contrast. It took an additional few weeks for my scan to get scheduled. I really wasn't too worried about it at the time.

The reason for the additional MRI that they gave me was that there was "an attenuation of gray and white matter in the right frontal lobe". Of course, not having a medical degree, or any real medical knowledge past watching Grey's Anatomy, I had no idea what that meant. In my google searching and asking around, I had come up with that it was probably something left over from an old sinus infection or possibly when I had covid-19 a few years before.

The morning of my MRI came. I wasn't really nervous. My mom worked at the hospital that I was getting my scan at. She met me down at check-in, more just to say hi since I lived so far away, and seeing each other was always a treat. My kids had the day off of school for the Easter holiday, so I did my scan, and immediately jumped back into the car to head back home to spend time with them. Not more than 30 minutes after making the trip back home, I got a phone call from the doctor asking if I was still in town. Of course, I wasn't. He said if I had been, a neurosurgeon could have made an exception to squeeze me in so I could have been seen that day. He then informed me that I had a mass in my right frontal lobe and needed to see a neurosurgeon to learn more about my condition.

I immediately began to panic. I called the surgeon to make an appointment as soon as possible. Since it was Friday, Monday was going to be the soonest I could get in. I had to go the entire weekend and through a family holiday pretending I was fine and nothing was wrong. I didn't have any real answers, and until I did, I didn't want to say anything. Of course my parents knew what was going on. I had to have an outlet of some kind other than crying in the bathroom for a few minutes before pulling myself back together. I didn't want to alarm my kids if it ended up not being a big deal.

Again, turning to google, I learned the word "mass" can mean many things. It does not immediately point to having a tumor, or even cancer. My family has always been a witty, sarcastic bunch. So, after my first scan, I started cracking jokes about what was growing in my head. The first being from the 80's movie "Twin's" "It's not a tumor" [in Arnold Scwarzenegger's voice]

I made it through the weekend and my mom went with me to my appointment. The surgeon that I first met with had been a longtime employee of the hospital. While still a neurosurgeon, this was not his usual type of procedure. It became quickly apparent that he was not the man for the job. Mom and I had discussed the possibility of this over the weekend, but it didn't matter to me either way, I wanted to see what was growing in my head. We could find the right person for the job after we knew what we were dealing with.

As previously mentioned, I had gone through a divorce. My ex carried the health insurance, so I had taken a part time job in the mornings at the UPS warehouse. It was going to take nine long months before I would qualify for health insurance, but I had my eye on the prize and I was determined to stick it out and make it work. It was the busy time of year at UPS and also at my salon. I was running myself ragged. My normally long days had now turned into 16 hour days six days a week. After a few months I started to not feel so great. I know what you're thinking, right? Duh, you can't keep that pace. That wasn't it though. I started to get dizzy, feeling nauseous, having constant headaches and pressure in my face, and the strangest nose bleeds. My daughter has had nose bleeds her entire life. These were not like that. I would have little blood clots come out when I blew my nose. I went to see my primary physician about it, and she explained to me that I could no longer put off the sinus surgery I was told I needed to have years before when I went to see an ear, nose and throat {ENT} doctor in Columbus. My doctor told me that if they did in-office cauterizing, she would do my entire nose. They didn't, so she had advised me not to even blow my nose or it would bleed.

I immediately got a hold of my mom and told her what was going on. She works at a hospital. She does credentialing and works closely with doctors, so she knows them on more of a personal level. I had resigned myself to needing to have sinus surgery, even though I was most definitely not looking forward to it. My mom recommended someone that she knew well and that she felt would do a good job. I made an appointment to drive the 2 hours one way to see him, since it would be closer to my parents. If I was going to have surgery I was going to need help and care.

My first appointment with the new ENT Dr. went ok, I thought. I told him everything that I had previously been told about needing sinus surgery, having a deviated septum and what not. He had asked if I could breathe through my nose, and I explained, kind of, through one side. I had always chalked it up to my deviated septum and allergies that I have. I also explained to him the pressure in my face, the bloody noses and the fact that I really couldn't smell anything anymore, unless it was very strong. He took an instrument that was long and skinny and looked up my nose. He then proceeded to tell me that he couldn't see any reason why I couldn't breathe. He said that there may be something that showed up on my CT inside my sinus cavity to explain what he couldn't see. He ordered a CT scan for me.

I made the trip back for the scan a couple of weeks later. I was at home when I got the call from the doctor that my scan was read by an Interventional Radiologist. He had seen a shadow and ordered an MRI, with and without contrast. It took an additional few weeks for my scan to get scheduled. I really wasn't too worried about it at the time.

The reason for the additional MRI that they gave me was that there was "an attenuation of gray and white matter in the right frontal lobe". Of course, not having a medical degree, or any real medical knowledge past watching Grey's Anatomy, I had no idea what that meant. In my google searching and asking around, I had come up with that it was probably something left over from an old sinus infection or possibly when I had covid-19 a few years before.

The morning of my MRI came. I wasn't really nervous. My mom worked at the hospital that I was getting my scan at. She met me down at check-in, more just to say hi since I lived so far away, and seeing each other was always a treat. My kids had the day off of school for the Easter holiday, so I did my scan, and immediately jumped back into the car to head back home to spend time with them. Not more than 30 minutes after making the trip back home, I got a phone call from the doctor asking if I was still in town. Of course, I wasn't. He said if I had been, a neurosurgeon could have made an exception to squeeze me in so I could have been seen that day. He then informed me that I had a mass in my right frontal lobe and needed to see a neurosurgeon to learn more about my condition.

I immediately began to panic. I called the surgeon to make an appointment as soon as possible. Since it was Friday, Monday was going to be the soonest I could get in. I had to go the entire weekend and through a family holiday pretending I was fine and nothing was wrong. I didn't have any real answers, and until I did, I didn't want to say anything. Of course my parents knew what was going on. I had to have an outlet of some kind other than crying in the bathroom for a few minutes before pulling myself back together. I didn't want to alarm my kids if it ended up not being a big deal.

Again, turning to google, I learned the word "mass" can mean many things. It does not immediately point to having a tumor, or even cancer. My family has always been a witty, sarcastic bunch. So, after my first scan, I started cracking jokes about what was growing in my head. The first being from the 80's movie "Twin's" "It's not a tumor" [in Arnold

Scwarzenegger's voice]

I made it through the weekend and my mom went with me to my appointment. The surgeon that I first met with had been a longtime employee of the hospital. While still a neurosurgeon, this was not his usual type of procedure. It became quickly apparent that he was not the man for the job. Mom and I had discussed the possibility of this over the weekend, but it didn't matter to me either way, I wanted to see what was growing in my head. We could find the right person for the job after we knew what we were dealing with.

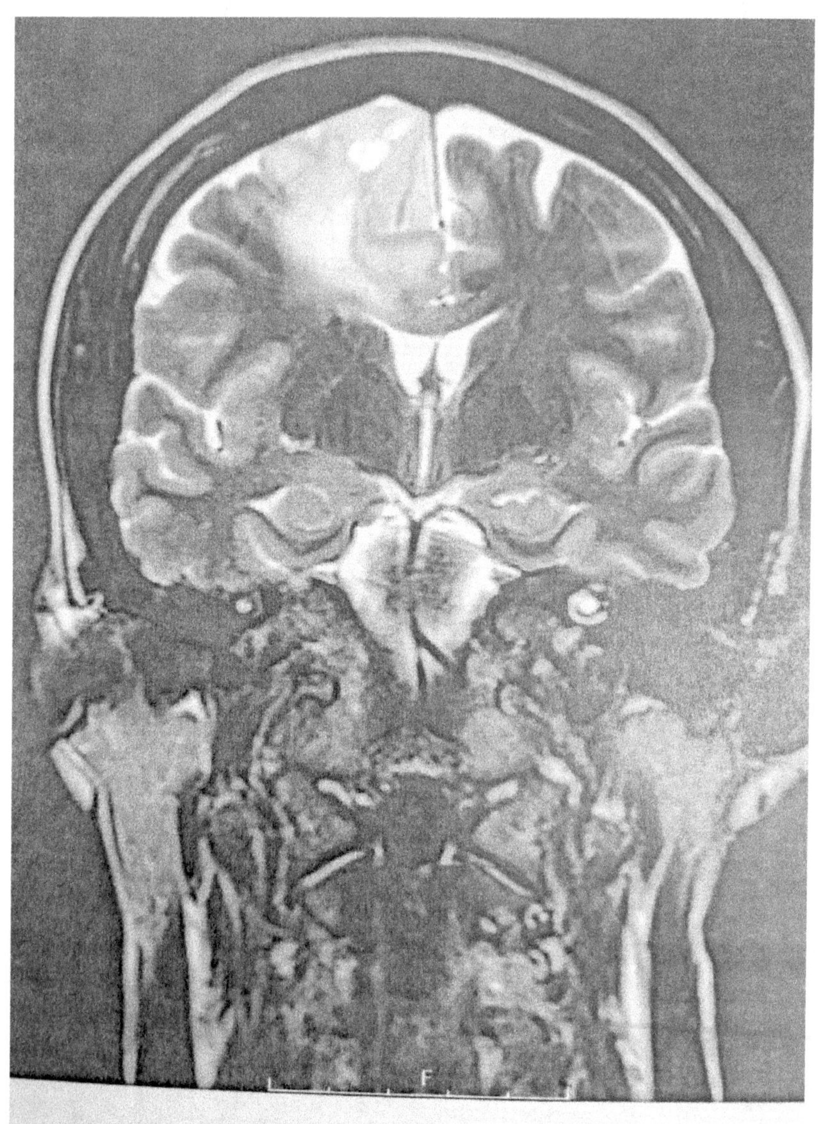

3

Surgery

After a few good recommendations, we narrowed down the right surgeon. I would be traveling the other direction in the state now. Omaha is the largest city in Nebraska. We are very lucky to have UNMC [University of Nebraska Medical Center] where many advancements are made in medicine regularly. This is not where I would find my surgeon though. I found my surgeon in a private practice close to Methodist Hospital.

In the beginning, it's already very difficult just to wrap your head around the fact that you have a tumor, then to find out that it's probably cancer. These people are the best of the best at what they do. They can usually tell with utmost certainty what it is that they are looking at.

My mom and dad went with me to my appointment. I had an introductory appointment with the surgeon to make sure that he was the one I wanted and that we all felt comfortable with. We all felt that he was very knowledgeable and took very seriously what he was doing. It was then that I got the first real picture of "Carl" my tumor. Of course, I named it.

I went back a few weeks later for a follow up appointment and to schedule surgery. At that point, I was told that surgery would take place before the end of May.

Insurance is wonderful, and believe me, I'm very thankful for having it, but sometimes having to jump through all of the loopholes can make a person want to pull their hair out!

I ended up having surgery on July 7th 2022 at Methodist Hospital in Omaha. I thought that I was ready. I thought I was tired of waiting and just wanted it over with, until it was right there..I have never been so scared of anything in my life! I was surrounded by my parents, kids, and my then boyfriend. I had even more come to visit me in the hospital while I was there over the next few days.

Let me tell you, brain surgery is not for the faint of heart! I remember waking up, seeing everyone and liking that they were there. Yet somehow, I did not have any emotions at all. My family was trying to laugh and joke with me, and I would just stare at them with a blank face. My internal dialogue thinking, I don't know why they're laughing, it's not funny.. I did remember having anger. I had a male nurse taking care of me. I had many nurses throughout my stay, but this one stuck out. He was absolutely great at his job, to the point of not letting me go to the bathroom by myself and I was not having it! He was standing in the doorway of the bathroom, watching me "try" to go. I felt the need to tell him that he needed to leave. Good guy that he was, he told me right back that I just had part of my brain removed and he wasn't leaving me alone. It's comical now to think about it. I'm not so sure he looks back on it quite as fondly.

I remember the first day being mostly nothingness and pain. I was very tired and slept a lot. The second day, I was starving, and ate the hospital's crappy breakfast like a champ! The eating kinda went downhill from there.

After a three or four day stay, I was released from the hospital, and allowed to go home with my parents. The ride home was not the most fun I've ever had, but it could have been much worse.

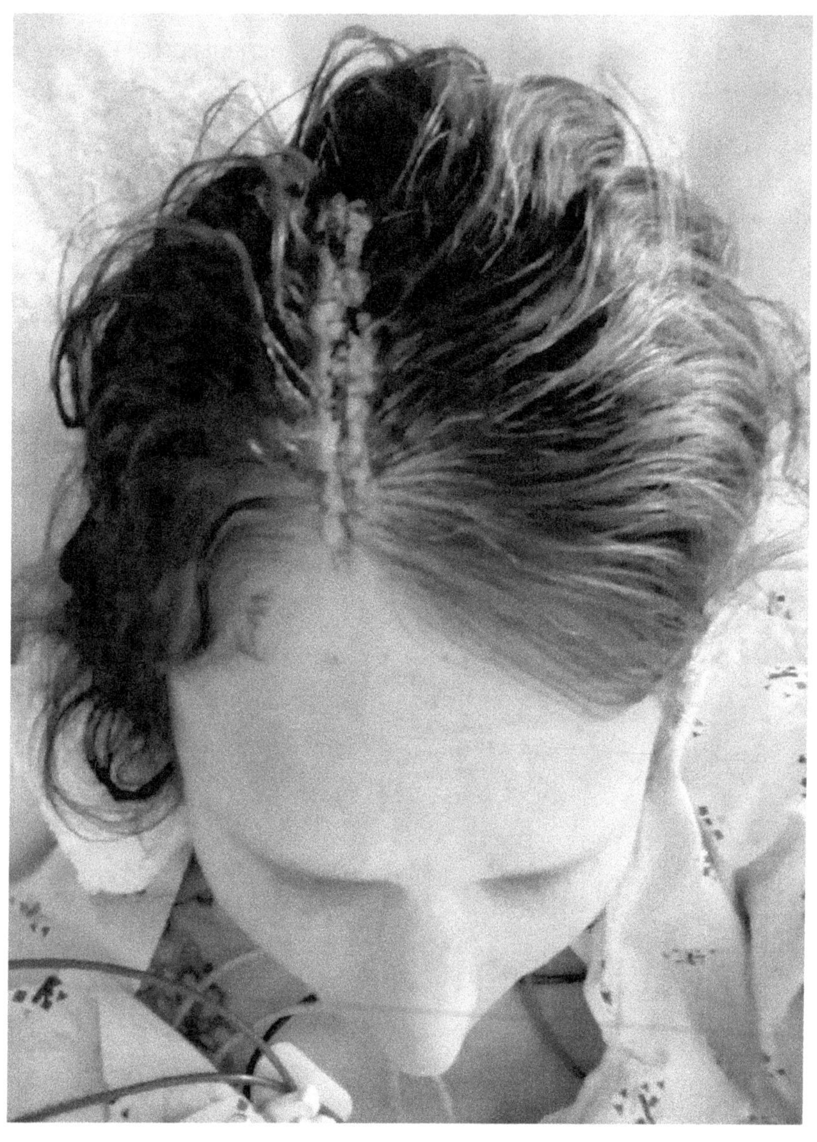

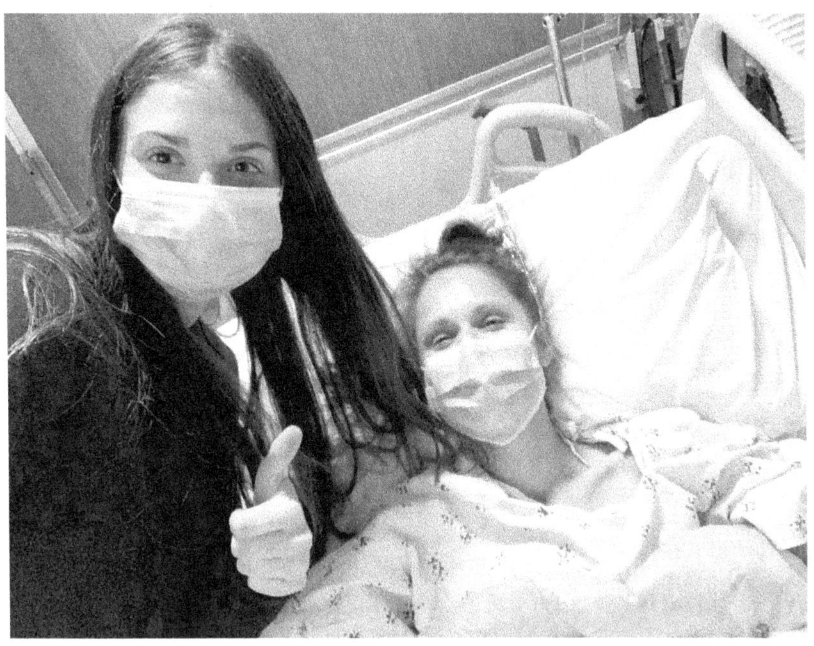

4

Recovery

At first I remember just being happy to be out of the hospital and in the comfort of my parent's home. I was mostly sleeping. My mom was staying with me round the clock keeping up with my med schedule and trying to force feed me like any good mother/caretaker. We had many jokes before surgery that we were going to do puzzles together for my neuroplasticity. Little did I know, she wasn't kidding. Most people would think brain surgery/puzzles, we should probably start small. Not my mom. She brought out the big guns right away. A 1000 piece puzzle! At first it was mostly just her. It made my head hurt just looking at it. Thinking had actually hurt at that point! It was like I could feel my brain carving a new path around the part that was now missing.

The puzzle became something of a force. I was drawn to it and loathed it at the same time. I can remember telling my mom that whoever created that puzzle was sadistic! I slowly was becoming a little more myself. Then one day I cracked up at something my mom said. "Oh good" she said, "I was worried you were going to have the emotions of a serial killer now." Apparently , at one point when the doctor came in to check on me, she asked if I was "normal." He assured her that it was just from the surgery and my body healing.

I was getting a little better each day. Baby steps. Then it hit. Swelling. Pain. Nausea. It was horrible! Nothing would touch it or take the edge off. Mom called the doctor's office and they called me on some steroids and anti-nausea meds to help combat what I was feeling. Let me tell you, I now understand why athletes take steroids! Holy cow! I felt great! Just like that, I could do almost anything by myself. I was still slow, and wore down quickly, but I felt AMAZING! We even went into town and went out to eat and watched all of the classic cars cruise around for cruise night. I had convinced myself, along with some help from those still at home, that I was ready to come home, I would be fine. WRONG. I could not have been more wrong. Sadly, what goes up [my steroid level] must come down. I spent the next few weeks at home on my couch in misery. I have been able to admit it for a while now, but it has never applied to anything more than this, I should have listened to my mother. She tried to tell me that I wasn't ready to go home yet, that it was too soon. Me being the stubborn person that I am, I wouldn't listen. I missed my kids, my animals and my house. Just being surrounded by my things. Dumb, dumb, dumb.

I missed my mom!. I missed someone cooking, taking care of me and being the adult. Now, I have to be the adult. Who made that decision? Oh wait, that was me. Simple things were hard. Things that always came second nature were gone. It seemed as though all of my thoughts were scattered, I was in pain constantly, and my body was not my own. Then came the phone call. Pathology had come back on "Carl". He was indeed cancerous. The big C word. It's one thing to "think" you know something, but it's something else to have it confirmed. That was a rough day. No more, maybe they're wrong. Nope. The only upside being, Carl had a genetic mutation that made him respond better to chemo. I was off work for a full 9 weeks recovering from surgery. Need to be caught up on a show? Just ask me, I'm sure I saw it. I had to promise that I would continue to do things for my brain and neuroplasticity once I was not being coerced by my mom. I had markers and an adult coloring book. I can't remember before that the last time I had colored a picture, My kids played Uno with me, and I had even bought a few puzzles of my own. It seemed that every puzzle I did by myself was unlocking some kind of achievement. In the weeks following, things became easier and easier. It wasn't as hard to do a simple task anymore. After 6 long weeks of being home, I finally got the OK from my surgeon to be able to drive. Freedom at last!

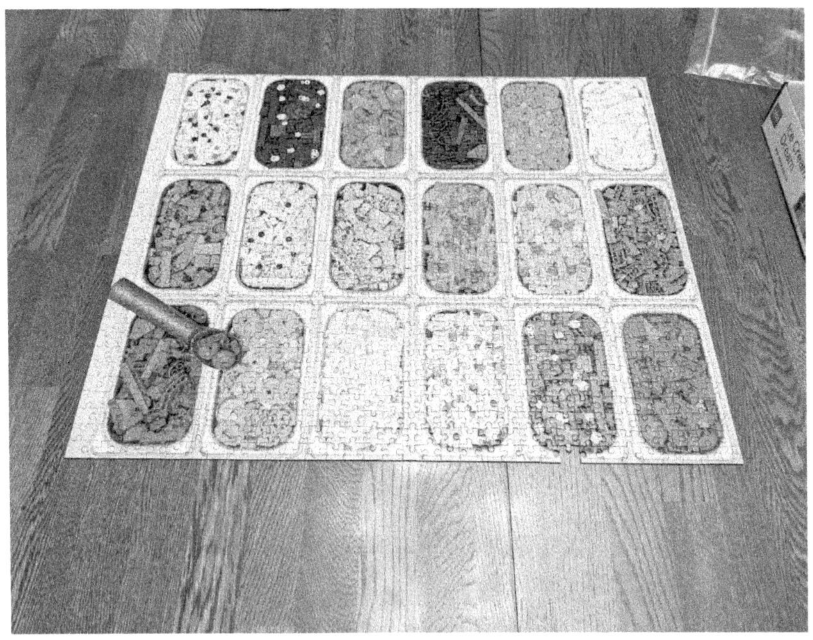

And yes, it was missing a piece!

5

Starting Treatments- Radiation

I started radiation treatments the Tuesday following Labor Day.. Again, mom came up for my first appointment. I have not gone one step alone through this process. She has been right there beside me. My battle buddy so to speak. We have cried together more times than I can count. I can't even imagine what it's like to have to see your child going through something like this. I can stay strong for my kids, because I think it makes it easier for them. I'm sure to some degree that is exactly what she's doing for me.

For anyone that has ever done radiation treatments, you know that they are not fun. Especially if you have a brain tumor. The oncology radiation team makes you a mask that conforms to your face and snaps it to the table so that you don't move. The treatments themselves do not take that long. Before every treatment they perform a mini CT just to make sure that it is all perfectly aligned. All in all, it's about 15 minutes beginning to end, at least mine were. The first few weeks I didn't feel any different. About Three weeks into treatments, My hair started to fall out around my temple area. Week four the area got bigger. I started to really feel the effects of the radiation. I chose not to work after my appointments, so that I could go home and take a nap if I needed to.

Weeks five and six, everything progressed. My hair fell out even more. I now looked like I had the reverse "ring" . I still had a chunk of hair over where my tumor was located [right on top of my head], but very little around it until right above my ears. As the weeks went on, I continued to lose hair.

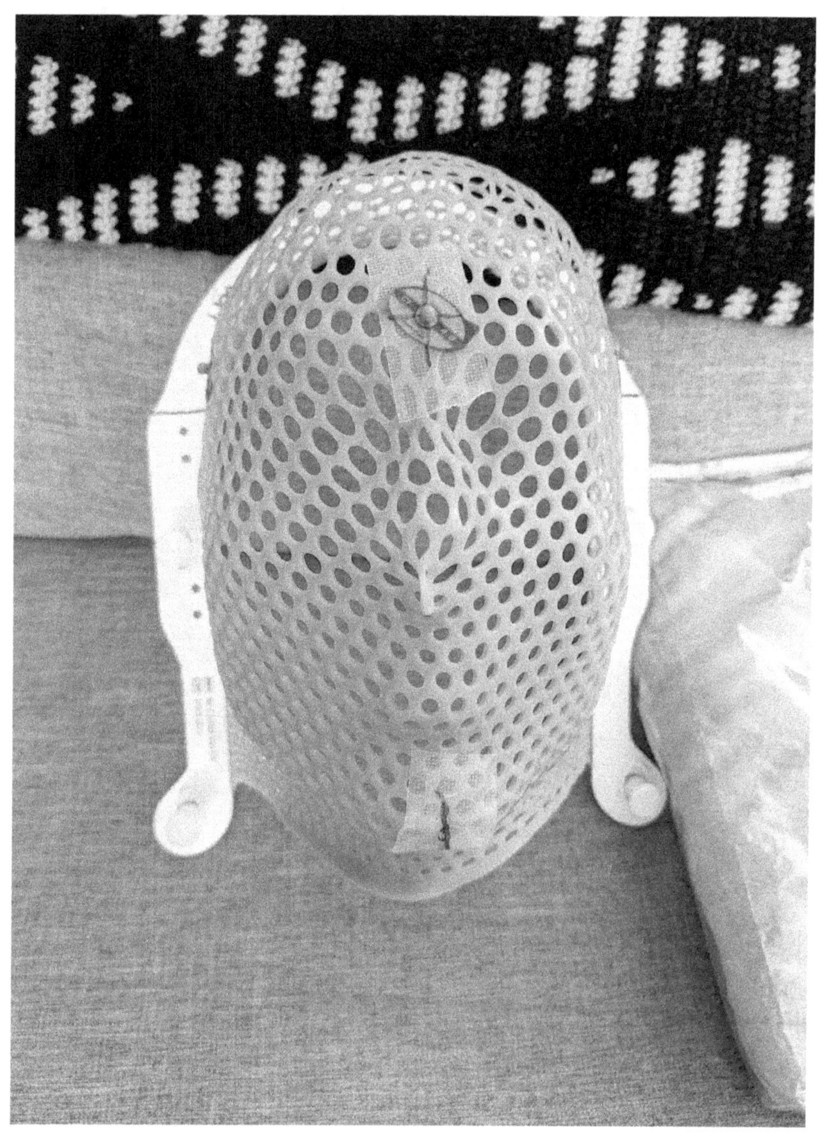

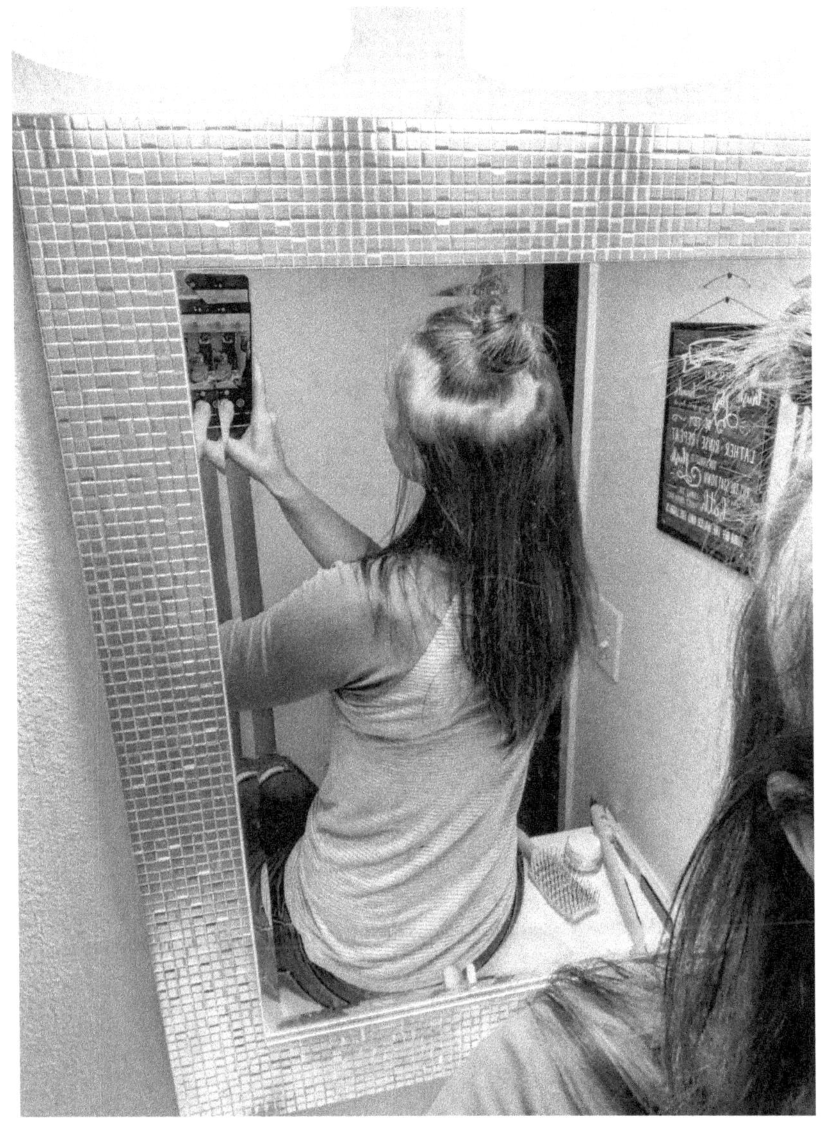

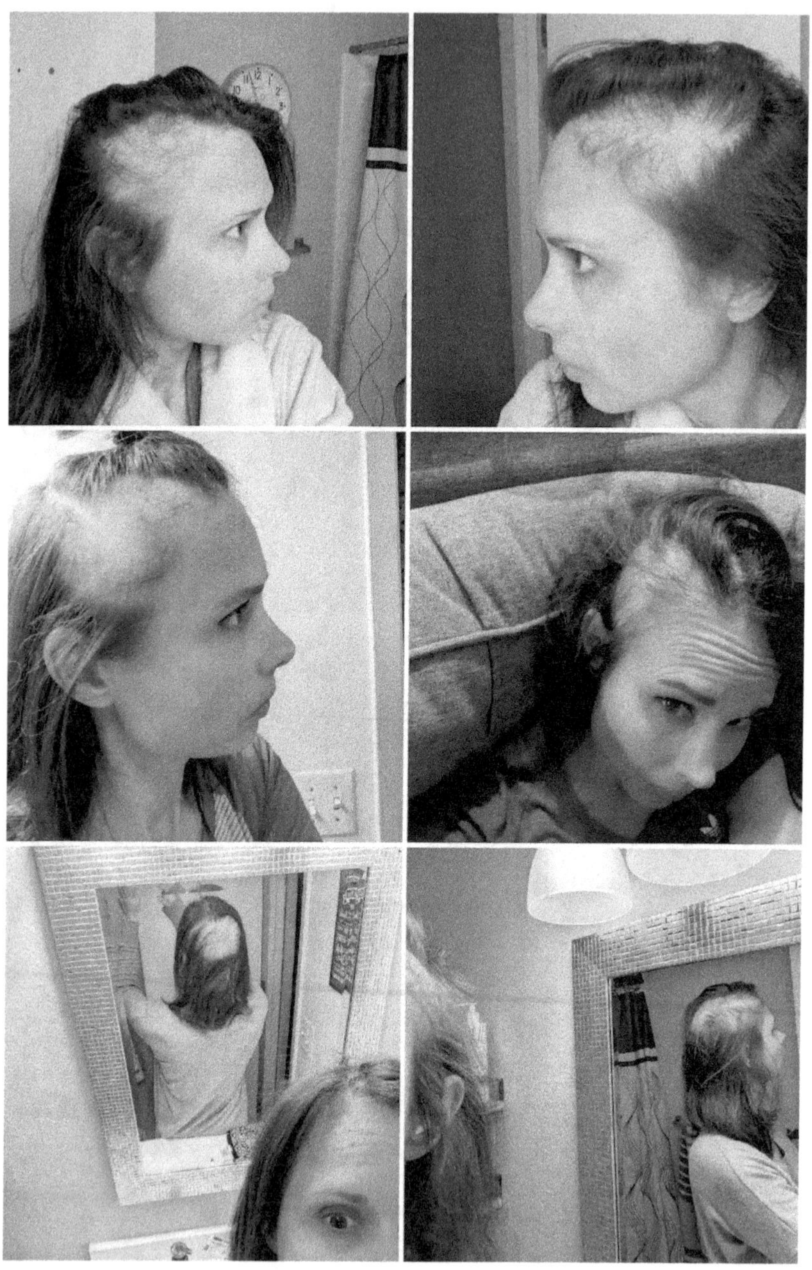

6

The In-Between

Before I had started radiation treatments, two of my best friends had decided that they were going to give me something to look forward to. They were taking me on a cruise!! A girl trip, when I finished radiation. I was so excited! I had six weeks in between my radiation and my chemo treatments. I had my hair packed and ready to go on vacation with me. And hats…lots of hats. I had the ok from all of my doctors, along with a list of things I could and could not do. Warm weather, the ocean, the beach, all of my favorite things. I had never been on a cruise before. It was an adventure and I had two of my best friends with me. We left for our trip three days after I finished radiation.

It was the most amazing 7 days! We had such a great time. All of the laughing at nothing, like you do with your best friends. You can just look at each other and crack up. We weren't even out of the airport yet and my sides and face hurt from laughing! They knew that I would be weak from treatment, so they had made arrangements ahead of time everywhere we went that I would have a wheelchair escort. Sometimes I used it, sometimes I didn't. It almost became a game of "who's name are they calling?' The days flew by. We spent our days at port on the beach, soaking up the sun and the sand. And the blended drinks. You can't go to the Caribbean without blended drinks. We have so many great memories from that trip. Jen and her gambling with Vanna, Shentell serenading us at dinner after drinking too much, while I was napping. Bingo in a giant room, Fabulous pictures, souvenirs, and weight gain. Holy food! Vacation stomach is definitely a thing. We decided that we should make it an annual trip.

The rest of my time off in-between radiation and chemo flew by. Before I knew it, it was

time for my oncology appointment.

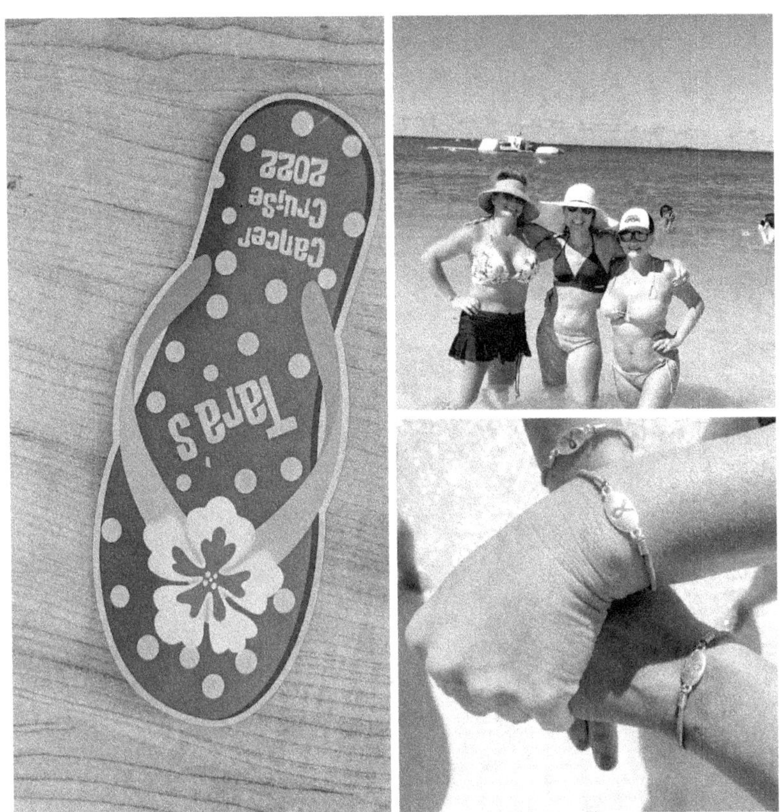
Cancer Cruise 2022
Tara's

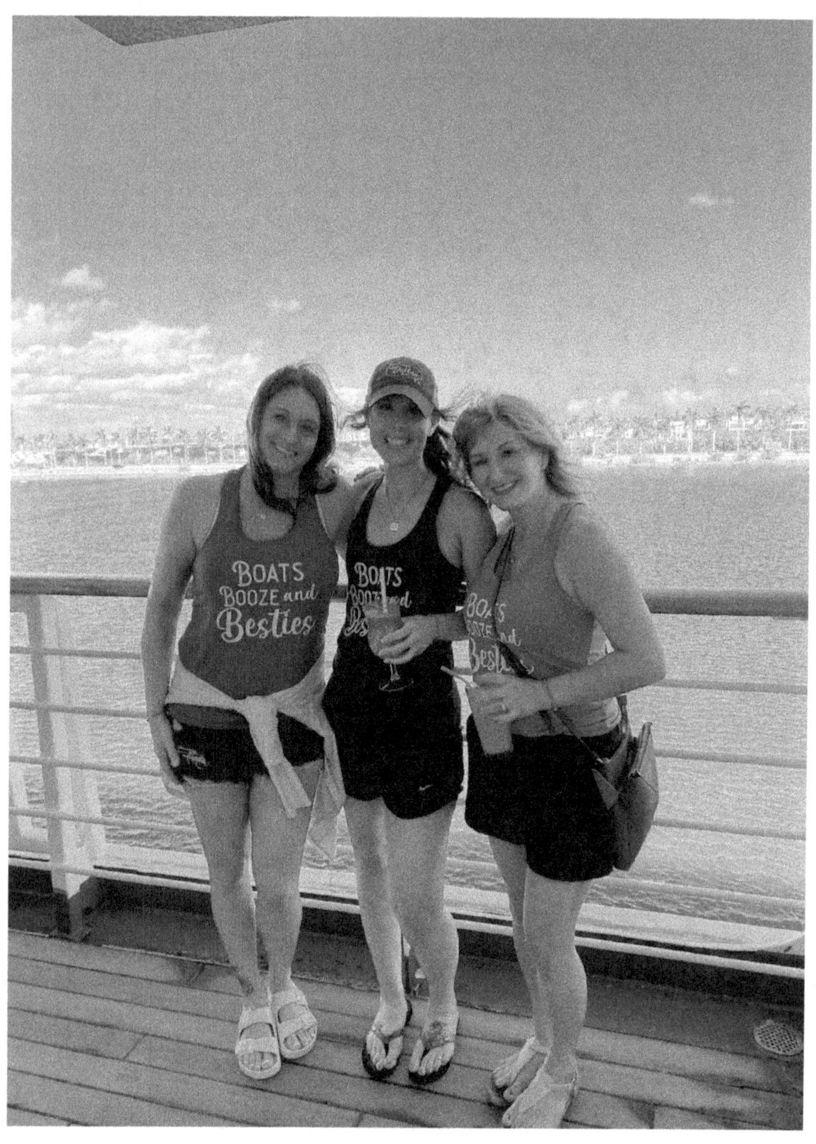

7

Treatments Continued-Chemo

The first time meeting my oncologist I was given so much information that it was hard to truly absorb it. I had had brain surgery a few weeks prior, and let's just say that I was not running at full capacity just yet. I looked fine to the casual observer, but to anyone looking closely or paying attention, they could notice the six inch scar running across my head, my balance issues, and me still struggling with nausea from too much motion.

I did not have a second oncology visit until I was done with my radiation treatments and my waiting period in-between them. This visit proved to be much more difficult. This was when I truly felt the gravity of my situation and it really started to sink in. Most people will not have a doctor sit them down and tell them that they need to prioritize their life, figure out what it is that they really want to do, and get on with it. Find out what is important to you. If you want to take a trip, do it. If you have a bucket list, now is the time to start crossing things off of said list. Once I was finished with my treatments, it was going to be "probably" the best few years that I have left. My tumor has a very high rate of recurrence, and as of today, my life span was 10 years. Also, in that 10 year span, expect for it to come back and we're going to do this all over again….unless there is a miracle, or medical advancements

. I know that medicine is changing every day, and I hold out hope that something will come about and they will start using the word cure. So far, in my oncology appointments, my doctor is very straightforward and consistently reminding me that "no detection" and "not currently growing" do not mean cured. It simply means it is laying dormant. The monster inside of my head is just "hibernating" for lack of a better term.

My oncologist was very optimistic the very first time that we spoke about my chemotherapy drug. I was actually relieved that it was going to be a pill, and not infusion therapy. I had heard horror stories from others about what chemo does to a person's body, life, job, etc. I had known people that had gone through it, but I was not part of the intimate circle to witness first hand what it was like. My relief was temporary. Do not be fooled, just because it is a pill, does not mean that there will be no side effects. It is not a "one size fits all" when it comes to how it will affect each person. It seems as though I was going to be one of the lucky few that got almost all of the listed side effects. Between feeling the effects of the chemo, making up for what I couldn't do while I was sick, and then seemingly catching everything around me, I was in a world of hurt my first few rounds.

From headaches, to body aches, nausea that just doesn't stop,hot flashes, being dizzy, having no appetite, then starving, and paying for it. The constipation….Oh lord, that is no joke! I have never spent more money on laxatives or consumed so many products to keep my system running in my life. To say the least, let's just say it doesn't paint a pretty picture.

I now have stomach issues, gas, bloating and a full-on mullet since my hair fell out around the top of my head. It has started to grow back a little. I no longer look bald anywhere. If you have ever had self esteem issues about your looks in the past, buckle up, they're about to go on overdrive! Most days anymore, I feel as though I'm walking around in someone else's body, and I want to crawl out of my skin. As a cosmetologist, I have always taken pride in my appearance and being put together, at least on the outside.Through this, I have never looked so awful for such long periods of time.It is a very humbling thing.

As I'm writing this, I'm getting ready to start my fourth of six rounds total. It feels as though I have been taking this drug for forever. It is winter right now, which does not exactly help. I believe very much in seasonal affective disorder. When the sun shines, I'm happy and full of energy. When it's gray and cloudy all day, well…the couch calls to me. I have also not been kind to my body being a hairdresser for 23 years. That takes its own toll on your body. I was falling apart before this honestly.

8

The Day to Day

As I have said previously, I feel very blessed to be surrounded by so many people that are in my corner cheering me on. Not only do I have my parents, which without them, I never would have made it through this, but my kids, friends, clients, and I live in a small community, so even people that I don't know have reached out to offer support. Not a day goes by that I don't have someone encouraging me and supporting me. I am very lucky in the aspect that my salon clients are also my friends. We have been in each other's lives for years, and genuinely care for each other. I feel as though I have an extended family, that should I ever need anything, all it would take is a phone call.

At the beginning when I came home, one of my friends set up a Go Fund Me account to help balance out the costs of daily life and still raising two teenagers. Their lives and needs do not stop because of my health issues. I had many more people that wanted to help out and sent money directly to me, my parents or my close friends. The kindness of strangers is truly amazing, and something I have a hard time wrapping my head around. Just when you feel that everything is bleak and sad, here come strangers to lend a helping hand! Not that I take for granted the people close to me, I do not. They are my safety, my support on the daily and the reason I can even have the strength to get through each day or get out of bed. It is very easy to think that there are no good people left in the world and that nobody cares. Get diagnosed and battle cancer in a small community, it will change that mindset completely. And not just my community, but where my parents live also. Support comes from all over! I still have people financially helping out that I have not even met. My mom will tell me, this is from my friend at work, or this is from my cousin that lives in another state.

I no longer wish that I could work the long days that I used to. My priorities have changed completely. I still work as much as I can, it just isn't quite the same as it used to be. I work far less hours now, because I physically can't do the workload that I used to, and even if I could I would choose not to. Not that my kids and family weren't a priority before, they always have been, but being diagnosed with a terminal disease and having a clock put on your life completely changes things. I no longer choose to work late nights, or weekends. Some of that is because right now my body just needs the time to recover. But I have made the decision that even after my treatments are done, I'm going to work less hours at the salon. My kids are in high school and I only have a few years left with them. I am going to make the absolute most of that time.

9

Doctors, Doctors, Doctors

I have so many different doctors these days, it seems as though my life is strung together from one doctor's appointment to another. From my neurosurgeon, to my radiation oncologist, my oncologist or my primary physician. And that doesn't count the MRI's every three months and the monthly blood work

Chemo takes a toll, and I feel as though I am forever taking this antibiotic or that one to fight a secondary infection.

Vitamins have also become a part of my everyday life. I used to go in spurts where I would take a multivitamin, then fall off, because I ran out and the bottle doesn't magically refill itself. I am now taking far better care of myself. My doctors have said "just be as healthy as possible". Applying that to someone that literally still ate like a kid, that wasn't overly helpful. I tend to be an all or nothing kind of person. I'm really good at being good for a while, and then I'll fall off and go back to my caffeine fueled, sugar laden ways.

Now that I have to check in with so many doctors on a regular basis, it has helped me to take stock in what I am actually putting in my body. Too bad I didn't do this years ago, I could have possibly saved myself a lot of trouble.

I have no idea what caused my tumor, nor do the doctors. Brain tumors are not genetic. Some of them have some genetic factors that can play into making you more susceptible to getting them, but that's as far as they can pinpoint for a cause.

10

My New Reality

As I have said before, I'm still going through treatments. With each passing day, I look more forward to June, when I will no longer be "going through" treatments and I will be finished with them. My days that are "good days" are now spent making big meals for my kids, working a full day at the salon, and cleaning my house like there's no tomorrow….because when I'm good I need to do whatever I can in the moment, I do not know what tomorrow will bring.

11

Dark Humor

The phrase "whatever gets you through it" has never been truer. When times get tough, you can't cry all of the time. Sometimes, you just need a good laugh, even if it's at the expense of yourself. If someone didn't know me, they would probably believe me to have a very bleak outlook on life. Of course I do at times. I allow myself little windows to let it all out [It isn't healthy to keep it all bottled up] and then I'm right back to cracking jokes. It is not the way that everyone would choose to process their grief, but this seems to be how mine comes out

We have all heard someone say, "If you want to hear God laugh, tell him your plan."

or "God will only give you what you can handle." In those two statements I would say, I have made many plans and none of them included cancer or a brain tumor, and also, God must think that I'm a badass to endure this after everything else I have already gone through in my life. I pray everyday for a miracle and for healing.

So as you can see, it has been a rollercoaster of a ride. There has been joy, tears, pain, sickness, sorrow and sometimes defeat...briefly. And also strength and triumph! I will not go quietly! I will go down fighting if that is the path I have to take. I will fight for all of the amazing people cheering me on and the ones praying for miracles. I'll fight to see the wonderful people my children grow up to be,their weddings and to see my grand babies. I am a fighter...

I hope that this can help in some way, even if it's just to know that you are not alone, and yes, someone else's life is messier than yours. My journey is not yet over, and hopefully won't be, for some time to come.

Thank you for reading my story. God Bless. Feel free to leave me a review.

About the Author